CUT YOUR CHOLESTEROL

An easy-to-follow guide to lower and manage your cholesterol — in just 12 weeks!

Dr Sarah Brewer

Quercus

CONTENTS

WHAT IS CHOLESTEROL?

Cholesterol is a fatty substance that's made in your liver from certain fats in your diet. A small amount is also obtained pre-formed from animal-based foods such as meat, egg yolks and prawns (shrimp).

Cholesterol acts as an important building block and is used to make:
- healthy cell membranes
- steroid hormones (such as cortisol, oestrogen, testosterone, progesterone)
- vitamin D
- bile acids
- Coenzyme Q10 – a vitamin-like substance essential for processing oxygen and generating energy within cells.

Chemical structure of cholesterol
$C_{27}H_{46}O$

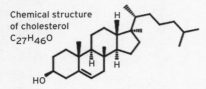

As cholesterol is so important, nature has even designed a special mechanism to stop you flushing too much down the loo. The only way to excrete cholesterol is via the liver into your bile. Bile is stored in your gallbladder, then squirted into your small intestines to help digest dietary fats. Almost all (97%) of the cholesterol reaching your gut in this way is absorbed straight back into your bloodstream, however, and sent back to the liver for processing. The only other significant way

- An adult weighing 150lb (68kg) has around 35g (1oz) of cholesterol.
- You make 800mg–1g cholesterol each day in your liver.
- You get 250–300mg pre-formed cholesterol from your food each day.
- Gallstones form when cholesterol crystallizes out from bile stored in your gallbladder.

to lose cholesterol from your body is to break it down and burn it as fuel.

So, a certain amount of cholesterol is vital for health. It's only when you make too much that the problem starts. Excess cholesterol clogs your arteries and increases your risk of coronary heart disease through a process known as atherosclerosis.

ATHEROSCLEROSIS When you make, or eat, too much cholesterol, the amount circulating in your bloodstream increases. If you lack antioxidants (which you get from eating vegetables and fruit) to protect this circulating fat, it undergoes a

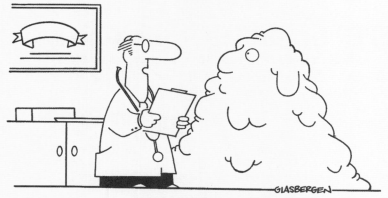

'You haven't been taking your
cholesterol medication, have you, Mr Smith?'

chemical reaction called oxidation. This is the equivalent of letting your cholesterol go rusty and rancid inside you.

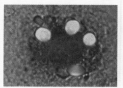

A macrophage foam cell containing fat droplets (shown in white)

Oxidized cholesterol is recognized as 'foreign' by scavenger cells (macrophages), which engulf it to form bloated 'foam' cells.

Foam cells try to leave your circulation by squeezing through the lining of your artery walls. Like an overweight person squeezing through a turnstile, they quickly become trapped due to their size. As they accumulate, they form fatty streaks along your artery walls.

It's a fact – fatty streaks are seen in the arteries of:
- 20% of children aged 2–15 years
- 60% of adults aged 26 years
- 70% of those aged 40

As these fatty deposits build up, they form raised plaques (atheroma) that make your arteries increasingly narrow. This hardening and furring-up of your arteries - known as atherosclerosis - leads to high blood pressure and increases your risk of heart attack and stroke.

CUT YOUR CHOLESTEROL

Over a quarter of all deaths from coronary heart disease could be prevented if everyone reduced their total blood cholesterol level by just 10%. And saving millions of lives is what this book is all about.

TYPES OF CHOLESTEROL

We need cholesterol to build and maintain our cell membranes, yet because it's insoluble, it can't simply travel around the body dissolved in the bloodstream.

Equally, it can't be allowed to float about in great lumps that would clog up your arteries. So your liver packages it into small parcels, ready to be transported, using special proteins that attract both fats and water. Within these spherical parcels, known as lipoproteins, the insoluble cholesterol stays on the inside, while the water-loving proteins remain on the outside. As a result, the packages become soluble when released into the circulation.

THE GOOD, THE BAD (AND THE UGLY)

There are two main types of cholesterol packages in your bloodstream. The main difference between these two types is in their relative size and weight.

Tests are available to measure the size of your circulating LDL-cholesterol particles. These are expensive, so are not yet widely available, although that may change in future.

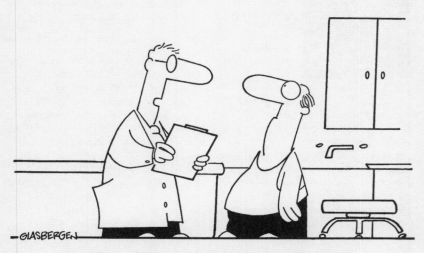

'No, HDL and LDL were not the robots in Star Wars.'

High-density lipoprotein (HDL)

High-density lipoprotein (HDL) cholesterol forms large, heavy particles that are too big to be engulfed by scavenger cells, or to seep into the artery walls. It's therefore referred to as 'good' cholesterol, as it stays in your bloodstream and helps to carry LDL-cholesterol back to the liver for processing. The good news: the higher your level of HDL-cholesterol, the lower your risk of cardiovascular disease.

Low-density lipoprotein (LDL)

Low-density lipoprotein (LDL) cholesterol is known as 'bad' cholesterol because its tiny, light particles can seep into the gaps between the cells lining your artery walls. It's also more prone to oxidation (damage by rogue free radical cells that leads to various diseases) and is readily engulfed by scavenger cells, which hastens atherosclerosis (a disease that narrows the arteries). Some people make very small, dense LDL-cholesterol particles and have an unusually high risk of developing coronary heart disease (CHD). Others make LDL particles closer in size to the gaps between the artery lining cells and have an intermediate risk of heart disease. The luckiest people make relatively large, less dense LDL-cholesterol particles and have a lower risk of heart disease. The size of your LDL particle depends partly on the genes you inherit, partly on your diet and lifestyle.

When it comes to atherosclerosis, it's the ratio of beneficial HDL to harmful LDL cholesterol that's the important factor:

TRIGLYCERIDES

Most fats in your diet (and in your body's fat stores) are in the form of triglycerides (see page 20). Your liver packages up triglycerides to be transported round the body as very low-density lipoprotein (VLDL) particles, which also contain some cholesterol. As the VLDLs pass through your circulation, the triglyceride component is removed and either burned as a fuel or stored as fat.

What remains becomes smaller and denser, and converts into 'bad' LDL-cholesterol particles. So, having a raised blood level of triglyceride VLDLs can also raise your cholesterol level, as well as increase your risk of cardiovascular disease. Ideally, if your triglycerides are raised, you want to bring them down to less than 1.7mmol/l (150mg/dl).

- If you have mostly HDL-cholesterol, your risk of CHD is significantly reduced.
- If your cholesterol is mostly in the form of LDL-cholesterol, your risk of CHD is greatly increased.

Research shows that for every 1% rise in your level of HDL-cholesterol, your risk of a heart attack falls by as much as 2%. This is due to something called 'reversed cholesterol transport' – put simply, HDL moves LDL-cholesterol away from your artery walls, back towards the liver.

WHAT RAISES CHOLESTEROL LEVELS?

Your blood cholesterol level is a balance between the amount of cholesterol released into your circulation by your liver, and the amount removed from your circulation by your body cells. So anything that raises the amount of cholesterol pushed out into your bloodstream, or that reduces the amount extracted from your blood, will cause your blood cholesterol levels to rise.

When a cell needs cholesterol it makes the necessary LDL-receptor cells and sends them to its surface, to act as fishing hooks. These receptors catch passing LDL particles and draw them inside the cell. On average, a particle of LDL-cholesterol circulates around your body for two and a half days until it's hooked into a cell; 70% of cholesterol removed from the circulation in this way is taken back up into the liver cells. If you have a good supply of circulating cholesterol, this will normally suppress your liver from producing new cholesterol.

HEREDITY The way your body handles cholesterol and other fats depends on your genes. You inherit two copies of each gene, one from your mother and one from your father. An estimated one in 500 people across the world possess a faulty copy of the gene that's needed to hook LDL-cholesterol into their cells (the LDL-receptor gene, see above). Even if these people also inherit a good copy of the gene from their other parent, their uptake of LDL-cholesterol is inefficient and these particles stay in their

circulation for longer than usual – typically, four and a half days. As a result, their cholesterol levels rise, leading to premature atherosclerosis and increased risk of heart attacks in their 30s and 40s. Over 1,000 different mutations in the LDL-receptor gene are known.

DIET Some people eat foods containing too much pre-formed cholesterol and saturated fats, increasing their LDL-cholesterol levels. If you inherit 'good' genes, your liver produces less LDL-cholesterol as your dietary cholesterol intake increases. 'Bad' genes, on the other hand, cause this negative feedback mechanism to malfunction, so your liver carries on churning out cholesterol even though you get plenty from your diet and have plenty in your circulation.

BEING OVERWEIGHT Carrying too much weight increases total and LDL-cholesterol levels while lowering your HDL-cholesterol – especially if you are apple- rather than pear-shaped. Having a beer belly (known as 'central obesity') is associated with something called insulin

Central obesity
(also known as 'having a beer belly')
is associated with insulin resistance,
which leads to cholesterol imbalances

resistance. When the muscle and fat cells no longer respond properly to insulin, glucose cannot enter the cells for use as fuel. This leads to all sorts of cholesterol-related problems. (For weight-loss tips, see also pages 30-31.)

LACK OF EXERCISE Regular exercise lowers 'bad' LDL-cholesterol while raising 'good' HDL-cholesterol - see pages 32-33.

THYROID FUNCTION One in ten people with a raised cholesterol level have an undiagnosed, underactive thyroid gland. Their slowed metabolism leads to a decline in cholesterol breakdown, although cholesterol production continues as normal. Proper treatment with thyroxine hormone can reduce cholesterol levels by as much as 40%.

If you haven't had your thyroid function tested in the past year, see your doctor — especially if you are lacking in energy and feel tired all the time. And take a trip to your doctor if you have abnormal cholesterol and/or triglyceride levels, and haven't had a kidney function test for 12 months.

KIDNEY FUNCTION Researchers have also found a link between long-term kidney disease, a high triglyceride level and a low HDL-cholesterol level.

RISK FACTORS FOR RAISED CHOLESTEROL

Some of us are more at risk of a raised cholesterol level than others. Doctors therefore screen those with the highest risk factors to help identify people whose cholesterol levels may lead to health problems in the future.

If you, or someone you know, is at risk of having a raised blood cholesterol level, your doctor will happily check this for you. Those who would particularly benefit from such screening include anyone who:

- Is aged 40 years or older (yes, really)
- Is younger than 40 but has a close family member (parent, brother or sister) who's experienced a premature heart attack or stroke (before the age of 55 years in men, and 65 years in women)

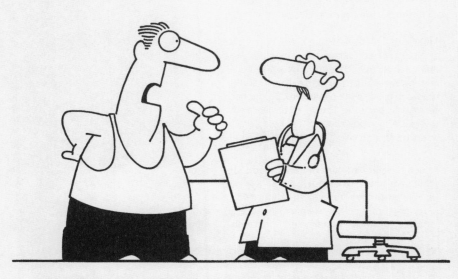

'I've always been a high achiever, always striving for bigger, faster, greater ... and now suddenly I'm expected to settle for lower blood pressure and less cholesterol.'

- Is overweight (especially if you store excess fat around your waist, see pages 8-9)
- Has a suspected family history of abnormally raised cholesterol levels (knowns as familial hyperlipidaemia)
- Has cardiovascular disease, including angina, heart attack, stroke, a type of mini-stroke known as a transient ischaemic attack (TIA) or peripheral vascular disease
- Has high blood pressure, diabetes or some other medical condition that can increase cholesterol levels, such as kidney or thyroid problems

SYMPTOMS AND SIGNS

The reason that doctors like to screen people for a raised cholesterol level is because there are few obvious symptoms or signs that can be spotted just by looking. A high cholesterol level does not usually cause symptoms until health problems such as angina, high blood pressure, heart attack or stroke develop. A few people might develop yellowish fatty lumps (xanthelasma) in the skin around their eyes, or fatty deposits (xanthoma) in the tendon sheaths around their knees, elbows, fingers or heels. Others may develop a premature yellow-white ring (arcus senilis) around the coloured part of their eyes (cornea) before the age of 40, but after this age, this may be a normal sign of ageing. These signs are usually obvious only in people who have inherited severe cholesterol-related problems, however.

KEEPING AN EYE ON YOUR OTHER RISK FACTORS

While lowering a high cholesterol level is important to reduce your risk of atherosclerosis, the development of heart disease involves many other risk factors to which you also need to pay attention – the more risk factors you have, the greater your chance of developing future health problems.

In fact, your doctor can predict your risk of developing coronary heart disease within the next ten years using special charts that include factors such as your age, gender, blood pressure, total cholesterol, HDL-cholesterol ratio and whether or not you have diabetes or smoke cigarettes.

Examples can be seen at the website: http://www.bhsoc.org/resources/prediction_chart.htm.

As well as checking your cholesterol level, your doctor will want to monitor your blood pressure, weight and glucose control. He or she may also want to assess your thyroid function, kidney function, homocysteine and CRP (though the last two are not routinely available on the NHS in the UK; see page 13).

> Make it a goal not only to have your cholesterol levels checked, but to become better acquainted with how your body works as a whole. You'll be able to recognize any health warnings or danger signs your body sends you and can act on them immediately.

TESTING

Blood-fat levels are measured first thing in the morning before you have had anything to eat or drink (that is, at 'fasting level'). Testing measures the total amount of cholesterol present, and how this is broken down into 'good' HDL- and 'bad' LDL-cholesterol particles; it usually assesses your triglyceride levels, too.

The unit used to measure blood levels of cholesterol and triglycerides is mmol/l – or millimoles per litre – in the UK; in the US, it is mg/dl – or milligrams per deciliter.

What counts as an acceptable level of cholesterol is not clear-cut and is regularly revised – usually downwards. In general, though, ideal levels are:

- total cholesterol of less than 5mmol/l (less than 200mg/dl)
- LDL-cholesterol of less than 3mmol/l (less than 100mg/dl)
- HDL greater than 1mmol/l (greater than 40mg/dl) for men, or 1.2mmol/l (greater than 50mg/dl) for women

You can assess your current total cholesterol level according to the following broad categories for the UK:
- ideal: less than 5mmol/l
- mildly high: between 5 and 6.4mmol/l
- moderately high: between 6.5 and 7.8mmol/l
- very high: above 7.8mmol/l

In the US, less than 200mg/dl is considered desirable; 200–239mg/dl is borderline high-risk; 240mg/dl and over is considered high-risk.

If other factors such as age, high blood pressure, having diabetes or being a smoker suggest that your risk of a heart attack is high, then your recommended total cholesterol level is even lower – below 4mmol/l – with your LDL-cholesterol ideally less than 2mmol/l. This usually means you'll be advised to take a cholesterol-lowering drug such as a statin (see pages 14-17).

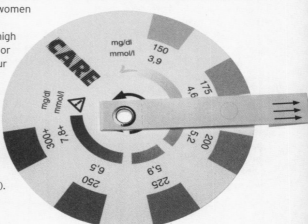

Ask your doctor what your target total cholesterol, HDL-cholesterol and LDL- cholesterol levels are and write them here:

MY TARGET total cholesterol level ·

MY TARGET HDL-cholesterol level ·

MY TARGET LDL-cholesterol level ·

OTHER TESTS Several other tests may be requested when your cholesterol levels are raised. These include thyroid function (see page 9), kidney function (see page 9), homocysteine and CRP (see below and box, bottom right).

Homocysteine is an amino acid that damages the artery walls and hastens atherosclerosis. People who have a high homocysteine level are at least three times more likely to have a heart attack than those with normal levels, and it appears to be as much of a risk factor for heart and circulatory problems as is LDL-cholesterol. Folic acid and vitamins B_6 and B_{12} supplements can lower homocysteine levels (see page 37).

C-reactive protein, or CRP, is a protein produced in the liver that can be used to indicate the level of inflammation in your body. Inflammation is linked with many diseases, including atherosclerosis. The CRP test appears to be twice as good at predicting the risk of a heart attack than a check of LDL-cholesterol. In fact, research suggests that half of all heart attacks and strokes occur in people who have acceptable cholesterol levels, but a high CRP level.

So, if you have borderline cholesterol or low HDL-cholesterol, or if you are at moderate risk of developing coronary heart disease due to other risk factors, this is a useful test. Statin drugs (see pages 14–17) used to lower raised cholesterol levels have been shown to reduce CRP levels.

It is not easy to have your CRP or homocysteine levels measured in the UK, as these tests are not yet routinely available on the NHS. They are available privately, however, if you are willing or able to pay for them.

MEDICAL TREATMENT

There are two main sources of cholesterol in your circulation – some is made in your liver (around 800mg per day) and some comes from your diet. If you have an abnormal cholesterol balance, your doctor may prescribe a type of drug called a statin.

Statin drugs target the liver's production of cholesterol by switching off the enzyme, HMG-CoA reductase, that is needed for it to be made.

The statin drugs licensed for use in the UK include: simvastatin, pravastatin, fluvastatin, atorvastatin and rosuvastatin. In the US, lovastatin is also available.

BENEFITS OF STATINS

Several large trials show that taking a statin for at least five years reduces the risk of coronary heart disease (CHD) by around a third and, for those who've already had a heart attack, it reduces overall death rates by approximately a quarter. Taking a statin also reduces the risk of a (non-haemorrhagic) stroke by up to 29% in those with CHD.

Initially, statins were prescribed for people with raised cholesterol levels. Then, in 2002, the Heart Protection Study, which involved over 20,000 people, showed that statins appeared to reduce the risk of major cardiovascular problems in everyone, even those with an ideal total cholesterol level of less than 5mmol/l.

Whether or not your doctor decides to prescribe a statin for you is therefore no longer based on your cholesterol levels alone. Statins are now recommended for anyone whose likelihood of developing CHD over the next ten years is 20% or greater, whatever their cholesterol level. This risk is calculated from charts, and is based on factors such as your gender, age, smoking status, blood pressure and whether or not you have diabetes – as well as your cholesterol level.

The general aim of treatment is to lower your LDL cholesterol to less than 3mmol/l and your total cholesterol to less than 5mmol/l, or by 30%, whichever is the greater. Some people at particularly high risk may have an even lower target set (see page 12).

The effectiveness of the treatment is reviewed after 4–12 weeks to see if you need to have the statin dose increased, or whether you may need to add in an additional treatment.

A blood test is also carried out to check for side effects in the liver or muscles (see the section on drawbacks, pages 16–17).

Trials show that taking a statin for at least five years reduces the risk of coronary heart disease (CHD) by around a third

OTHER DRUGS A drug known as a cholesterol absorption inhibitor (ezetimibe) works by blocking the absorption of cholesterol from the intestines. Ezetimibe is used together with a statin, so both the production of cholesterol in the liver and its absorption from the intestines are reduced. This is efficient in bringing down high cholesterol levels in 72% of people who are unable to reach their target cholesterol levels by taking a statin drug alone.

Older drugs such as bile acid sequestrants (eg colestyramine), anion-exchange resins (eg colestipol) and fibrates (eg bezafibrate) are now rarely used to lower cholesterol alone, unless the person has very high levels that do not respond to a maximum dose of a statin plus ezetimibe. A fibrate drug may be used along with a statin if triglyceride levels remain high. Or nicotinic acid (vitamin B_3) may be used to lower stubborn triglyceride or LDL-cholesterol levels further.

THE DRAWBACKS OF STATIN
TREATMENT

Like all drugs, statins have the potential to cause side effects such as headache, nausea and bowel disturbances. In addition, 1 – 5% of people taking a statin may develop muscle problems such as pain, inflammation and weakness.

WARNING: If you are taking a statin, tell your doctor promptly if you develop unexplained muscle pain or any tenderness or weakness. If muscle problems (myopathy) occur, treatment will be stopped if the symptoms are severe, or if your blood levels of a muscle enzyme, creatine kinase, rise significantly.

Out of every 100,000 people taking a statin for a year, at least one person will also develop a rare condition called rhabdomyolysis, in which the muscle fibres break down. If this affects the heart, it is obviously serious, but muscle pigments (myoglobin) entering the circulation can also damage the kidneys.

As well as switching off cholesterol production in the liver, statins also switch off production of a substance called

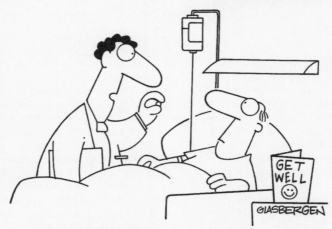

'We found a bunch of these clogging your arteries.
They're cholesterol pills.'

All statins sold in Canada are required to carry a warning that they may seriously deplete Coenzyme Q10 levels in the body, which can lead to impaired heart function in people with congestive heart failure. Taking a Coenzyme Q10 supplement is especially important for those on statins who have familial hypercholesterolaemia (inherited raised cholesterol levels), heart failure or who are over 65 years of age. Research confirms that combining a statin drug with 60mg Coenzyme Q10 improves the heath benefits to your heart, compared with taking the statin alone.

Coenzyme Q10, which contributes to these muscle problems. Statins reduce Coenzyme Q10 levels by a similar amount to the reduction in cholesterol (40-50%), but often do so more quickly. In fact, taking a statin can halve circulating levels of this substance within just two weeks.

Coenzyme Q10 is needed for energy production in all of the body cells, especially the muscle cells. Although lowering levels of Coenzyme Q10 may not cause problems for healthy volunteers, it worsens heart problems in some people. Biopsies from people with various forms of heart disease have shown, for example, that between half and three-quarters are deficient in this vitamin-like substance.

Taking Coenzyme Q10 supplements helps to maintain blood levels of Coenzyme Q10 without affecting the cholesterol-lowering effect of statin drugs.

VITAMIN E A less well-known fact is that statins also lower blood levels of vitamin E by 17%. As vitamin E is vital in protecting against free radicals, this means LDL-cholesterol is more likely to become damaged and involved in the onset of atherosclerosis. If you are taking a statin, it's worth ensuring that your supplement regime also includes vitamin E – ideally along with other antioxidants that work with it, such as vitamin C, selenium, carotenoids (see pages 36-39), alpha-lipoic acid and l-carnitine.

Statins are effective drugs as long as you are aware of their drawbacks. To help reduce the dose you need (and to reduce your risk of side effects) your doctor will also provide diet and lifestyle advice to complement your medication. The information in the following pages provides detailed information to help wash cholesterol out of your system.

WARNING: Grapefruit juice interacts with statin drugs to increase their levels in the blood. For example, taking one particular statin (lovastatin) with a glass of grapefruit juice produces the same blood levels of the drug as if you had taken 12 tablets with water! If you are taking medication, check the drug information sheet provided for grapefruit interactions.

LOWERING CHOLESTEROL BY DIET

There are two main sources of cholesterol – some is obtained pre-formed in your diet from animal sources (around 300mg per day) and some is made in your liver from dietary saturated fats (around 800mg per day).

Paying attention to your diet has an impact on both of these sources, and can lower your total and LDL-cholesterol levels, lower your triglycerides, raise your HDL-cholesterol and reduce your risk of atherosclerosis, heart attack and stroke.

In 2003, scientists from London and New Zealand came up with the concept of a Polypill; containing a cocktail of six different drugs, it had the potential to reduce cardiovascular disease by a massive 80% by lowering cholesterol, blood pressure and blood stickiness.

In an interesting twist, a group of scientists from Belgium, Australia and the Netherlands designed a Polymeal to produce the same beneficial effects through diet alone. Their research, published in the *British Medical Journal* in 2004, suggests that eating just seven superfoods can reduce your risk of a heart attack or stroke by a similar amount (76%). They predicted that eating these foods on a daily basis (fish two to four times per week) can increase life expectancy by six and a half years for men, and five years for women. From nutrition alone!

> The six drugs suggested for the Polypill were: a statin, three blood pressure-lowering drugs (a thiazide, a beta blocker and an ACE inhibitor), folic acid and a mini-aspirin.

THE SEVEN SUPERFOODS they suggest you eat regularly are:

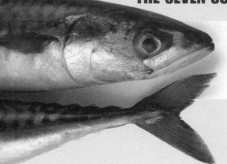

FISH – one portion (115g/4oz) four times a week reduces heart disease due to the omega-3 fatty acids that thin the blood and stop abnormal heart rhythms.

FRUIT AND VEGETABLES (excluding potatoes) – 400g/14oz daily (at least five servings) reduces blood pressure due to the antioxidant content.

ALMONDS – a handful (70g/2.5oz) per day significantly lowers total cholesterol levels due to the monounsaturated fats present in almond oil.

GARLIC – two to three cloves every day may not win you any friends, but garlic is a source of allicin, a substance that lowers cholesterol, reduces high blood pressure and makes the arteries more elastic.

A DAILY GLASS OF WINE (150ml/5fl oz) cuts your risk of coronary heart disease due to its high antioxidant levels. Although the scientists did not specify what colour of wine to drink, research suggests that the antioxidants found in red wine make it superior to white wine.

Although wine is often considered a health no-no, omitting the daily glass of wine had the strongest negative effect on the so-called Polymeal's beneficial effects, lowering the reduction in heart disease risk from 76% to just 65%.

DARK CHOCOLATE – yes, chocolate! Enjoying 100g/3.5oz dark chocolate per day (one small bar) can lower your blood pressure even more than fruit and vegetables. Chocolate is a rich source of the same type of antioxidant polyphenols that give red wine and green tea their heart-friendly reputations.

Surprisingly, olive oil was not included in the Polymeal, as the researchers did not find enough solid evidence to support it as a single ingredient rather than as part of the Mediterranean diet!

CURBING PRE-FORMED CHOLESTEROL

Reducing the average total blood cholesterol level by 10% could prevent over a quarter of all deaths from coronary heart disease. This is not the same as reducing dietary cholesterol intake, however. Read on ...

When you have raised LDL-cholesterol, you can still eat foods containing pre-formed cholesterol as long as you eat them in moderation. Studies show that, in most people, these foods raise LDL-cholesterol levels only minimally, while providing health benefits in the form of antioxidants, lecithin (see page 38) and important trace minerals.

While eggs were once scorned, research involving over 100,000 men and women shows that eating one egg a day does not increase the risk of coronary heart disease or stroke – even if your cholesterol level is raised. The best advice is to limit your cholesterol intake to no more than 300mg per day, which is about the amount found in one egg yolk. (Some people with a very raised cholesterol level may be advised to limit their intake to 200mg per day.)

STEWING OVER SATURATED FATS

It helps to know a bit more about what fat is. The fats in your diet consist of a molecule of glycerol from which three fatty-acid chains are attached to form a molecular shape similar to a capital E.

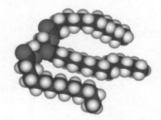

These are known as triglycerides.

The fatty-acid chains are of three main types. Those containing no double bonds are referred to as saturated fatty acids (SFA), those with one double bond are monounsaturated fatty acids (MUFA, see page 25) and those with two or more double bonds are polyunsaturated fatty acids (PUFA, see pages 22–23).

Most dietary fats contain a blend of SFA, MUFA and PUFA in varying proportions. One type of fatty acid

WHEN BUYING EGGS, SELECT THOSE THAT ARE OMEGA-3-ENRICHED

generally predominates and the fat is classified on that basis. Although animal fats are classed as saturated fats, however, even lard and beef dripping contain more beneficial monounsaturated fats than harmful saturated fats! The fat found in steak is typically 51% monounsaturated, 45% saturated and 4% polyunsaturated. Not a lot of people know this.

Grams per 100g in red meat

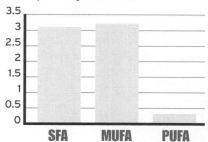

Although some dietary saturated fats are converted into cholesterol in the liver, over a third of those found in meat and dairy products have a neutral effect on your cholesterol levels. This does not mean that a high saturated fat intake is harmless, however. Like all types of fat, it has a high calorie content and excess is linked with obesity. And, if you have a high cholesterol level, you may have inherited genes that mean you process saturated fat less well than other people.

Ideally, saturated fats should supply no more than 7-10% of your energy intake, which, for most people, means cutting back. Replace them with more beneficial fats – the omega-3s (see pages 22-23) and monounsaturates (see pages 24-25).

The table below highlights some foods with a relatively high cholesterol content – eat those at the top especially in moderation.

SOURCE	Cholesterol/100g
Pig's liver	700mg
Lamb's kidney	610mg
Caviar	588mg
Lamb's liver	400mg
Chicken liver	350mg
Calf's liver	330mg
Margarine	285mg
Prawns (shrimp)	280mg
Sheep's tongue	270mg
Lamb's heart	260mg
Pheasant meat	220mg
Butter	213mg
Squid	200mg
Whelks	125mg
Duck meat	115mg
Lobster	110mg
Chicken (dark meat)	105mg
Red meat	100mg
Hard cheese	100mg
Mussels	58mg
Chicken (white meat)	70mg

MINDING YOUR OMEGA-6s AND OMEGA-3s

Here's the science: unlike saturated fats, polyunsaturated fatty acids (PUFAs) have a molecular structure that contains double bonds, in which hydrogen atoms are missing. If the first double bond is in position 6 on the molecule, they are called omega-6s, and if the first double bond appears in position 3, they are known as omega-3s.

Omega-6s are mainly derived from vegetable oils such as sunflower, safflower and corn oils, while omega-3s are mainly obtained from fish oils, having originally come from the plankton on which they feed. Your body handles omega-3 and omega-6 oils in different ways.

OMEGA-3S – THE GOOD GUYS

Overall, omega-3s have a neutral effect on LDL- and HDL-cholesterol levels, or may slightly raise good HDL and slightly lower LDL with no change in total cholesterol (it depends on the genes you've inherited). The other beneficial effects of fish oils make them vital for people with a raised cholesterol level, however. Omega-3s reduce inflammation – and remember, atherosclerosis is now recognized as an inflammatory condition. They also reduce blood stickiness to prevent unwanted clotting, significantly lower triglyceride levels (by up to 50%) and reduce abnormal heart rhythms. The protective effects of consuming fish oils develop within four weeks of increasing consumption and continue to improve so that, after two years, those on a high-fish diet are almost a third less likely to die from coronary heart disease than those eating very little fish. Eating fish two to four times a week lowers your risk of a stroke by over a quarter, while eating fish five or more times a week can reduce the risk of a stroke by more than half (though see page 43).

OMEGA-6S – GOOD IN MODERATION

When you eat a balanced amount of omega-6s, although they reduce total and LDL-cholesterol, they also lower HDL-cholesterol. Most people have too many omega-6s in their diet (from margarines, spreads, processed and ready meals), which promotes inflammation. Excess omega-6s are also susceptible to oxidation damage. Oxidation of omega-6 fats forms lipid peroxides, which are especially harmful, and contribute to atherosclerosis (see box, opposite).

The average Western diet currently contains a ratio of omega-6 to omega-3 fats of around 7:1, which is far too high.

Ideally, the balance between these two types of fats should be no more than 3:1. This means that most people should cut back on the types of food that contain omega-6s and increase their intake of foods that contain omega-3s. In fact, human beings evolved on a Stone-Age, hunter-gatherer diet of green plants, wild animals and fish that contained equal amounts of omega-6s (from natural vegetable oils) and omega-3s (from oily fish) – a ratio of 1:1.

To cut out excess omega-6s, eat fewer:

- vegetable oils
- margarines
- convenience and fast foods
- manufactured goods such as cakes, sweets and pastries.

TO REDUCE FORMATION OF TOXIC LIPID PEROXIDES:

- Don't eat excessive amounts of omega-6 fats
- Eat lots of fruit and veg – dietary antioxidants protect against harmful oxidation
- Don't overheat oils so they smoke while cooking
- Don't reuse oils over and over again

THE OILY FISH INCLUDE:

- Anchovy (unsalted)
- Bloater
- Carp
- Eel
- Herring
- Hilsa
- Jack fish
- Kipper
- Mackerel
- Orange roughy
- Panga
- Pilchard
- Salmon
- Sardine
- Sprat
- Swordfish
- Trout
- Tuna (fresh, but not tinned)
- Whitebait

Eat at least two portions of these a week – but don't deep-fry them or smother them in salt. Grill 'em or bake 'em!

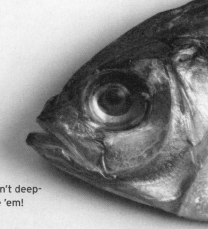

MAJORING ON MONOUNSATURATED FATS

More science: monounsaturated fats consist of chains of carbon atoms in which there is only one double bond, making it nice and flexible.

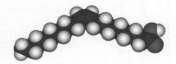

Your body deals with monounsaturated fats in such a way that they lower LDL-cholesterol levels with no effect on HDL levels. They also improve insulin sensitivity, which helps your body handle glucose. A diet high in monounsaturates may help to reduce your risk of atherosclerosis, high blood pressure, coronary heart disease, stroke and type 2 diabetes. This is thought to explain some of the benefits of the so-called Mediterranean diet. Foods rich in monounsaturates include avocados, olive oil, rapeseed (canola) oil and certain nut oils.

A diet rich in monounsaturates such as olive oil reduces the risk of coronary heart disease by 25% and the risk of a second heart attack by 56%.

TYPE OF OIL	% monounsaturated fat	% saturated fat
Hazelnut oil	82%	7%
Macadamia nut oil	81%	13%
Olive oil	73%	14%
Rapeseed oil	60%	7%
Almond oil	68%	5%
Avocado oil	62%	12%
Peanut oil	44%	20%

Eat a handful of monounsaturate-rich nuts per day, use olive oil for cooking, and hazelnut, macadamia nut or avocado oil in salad dressings.

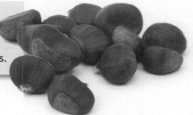

RESEARCH FINDINGS

- Eating a handful of almonds per day (about 23 kernels) can lower LDL-cholesterol by 4-5% and increase HDL-cholesterol by 6%.
- Eating an avocado a day can increase beneficial HDL-cholesterol by 11% within a week.
- Eating 85g/3oz walnuts daily for four weeks can reduce LDL-cholesterol by 16%.
- Eating a handful of macadamia nuts a day for four weeks can lower total and LDL-cholesterol by 5%. There were also positive effects on beneficial HDL-cholesterol levels.

TRASHING TRANS FATS Trans fatty acids are the most dangerous type of dietary fat for anyone, especially those with a raised cholesterol level. Trans fats are formed artificially when monounsaturated and polyunsaturated oils are partially hydrogenated to solidify them. This produces trans fats whose molecular structure twists around on itself so they can't slide nicely over one another. As a result, they form a tangled, solid mess at room temperature – just what manufacturers want when turning cheap vegetable oils into margarine.

Trans fats are bad to eat because they increase the activity of an enzyme (cholesteryl ester transfer protein) that raises LDL-cholesterol and lowers HDL. In addition, they become incorporated into cell membranes to increase their rigidity.

Research shows a strong link between consumption of trans fats and increased risk of coronary heart disease. Those with the highest intake have a 50% greater risk of a heart attack compared to those with the lowest intake. Trans fats are also linked with the development of certain cancers, including those of the breast and prostate gland.

Because of health worries regarding trans fats, nowadays margarines and low-fat spreads are being reformulated to reduce their trans fat content. Many processed foods do still contain high amounts of trans fats, however. Guidelines suggest reducing your intake of trans fatty acids to no more than 2% of your total energy intake. These guys are much more harmful to your health than saturated fats. So beware!

Start to pay more attention to what's in your food before you buy. Take time to check the labels, and select products that contain the lowest amounts of trans fats or partially hydrogenated polyunsaturated fats.

GETTING YOUR FIVE-A-DAY
Many nutritionists now believe that coronary heart disease is not so much linked to a high saturated fat intake, but to a lack of the dietary antioxidants that protect circulating fats from oxidation.

Rather than advocating the usual low-cholesterol, low-saturated-fat diet (which can also lower good HDL-cholesterol), they recommend increasing your intake of fruit and vegetables. These are a rich source of antioxidants, vitamins, minerals, fibre (see pages 28-29), isoflavones (see page 38) and other beneficial plant substances (phytonutrients). Polyphenols in red wine, blueberries and green tea, for example, have an effect on nitric oxide, a chemical that plays a role in the development of cardiovascular disease.

Research from Harvard University involving over 126,000 people shows that, even after taking other heart-disease risk factors into account, those with the highest intake of fruit and vegetables were 20% less likely to have a heart attack over the next decade compared with those eating the least. Each additional serving of fruit or vegetables eaten per day reduced the risk of coronary heart disease by 4%. And another large study of almost a quarter of a million people showed that stroke risk fell, too.

EACH OF THESE PROVIDES ONE SERVING:

- A whole apple, orange, pear, peach, kiwi, banana or similar-sized fruit
- A couple of satsumas, plums, apricots, figs, tomatoes or similar, smaller fruits
- Half a grapefruit, guava, mango, Galia melon, avocado
- A handful of grapes, cherries, blueberries, strawberries, dates etc.
- A tablespoon of dried fruit such as raisins or cranberries
- A handful of chopped vegetables/ pulses such as cabbage, sweetcorn, carrots, broccoli, beans, lentils, chickpeas

- A small bowl of mixed salad leaves
- A small bowl of vegetable soup
- A wine glass (100ml/3.5fl oz) of fruit or vegetable juice (these count towards a maximum of one serving per day only, as they don't contain much fibre)

TIP: A smoothie made by liquidizing whole fruit can count as more than one portion – measure the amount of fruit going into the container.

NOTE: potatoes do not count towards your vegetable servings as they consist mainly of starch. More flavoursome sweet potatoes do count, however.

ORAC: WHAT'S THE SCORE?

The antioxidant potential of fruit and veg is assessed by measuring their ORAC (Oxygen Radical Absorbance Capacity) score. Based on surveys in the US, scientists estimate that the average person gets around 5,700 ORAC units per day. Ideally, you need at least 7,000 for health; the optimum level to aim for if you have raised cholesterol is 20,000 units per day, or more. The following table lists foods and their ORAC scores.

Foods per 100g (3.5oz) and their ORAC scores

Food	Score	Food	Score
Dark chocolate	103,971	Peanuts	3,166
Pecan nuts	17,940	Red cabbage	3,146
Red kidney beans	14,413	Raisins	3,037
Walnuts	13,541	Gala apples	2,828
Pinto beans	12,359	Beetroot	2,774
Pomegranates	10,500	Golden Delicious apples	2,670
Red lentils	9,766	Spinach	2640
Hazelnuts	9,645	Aubergines (eggplants)	2,533
Cranberries	9,456	Lemons/Limes	2,412
Blueberries	9,260	Avocados	1,933
Prunes	8,578	Pears (green varieties)	1,911
Black beans	8,040	Oranges (navel)	1,814
Pistachios	7,983	Peaches	1,863
Black plums	7,339	Red leaf lettuces	1,785
Globe artichokes	6,552	Pears (Red Anjou)	1,773
Red plums	6,239	Macadamia nuts	1,695
Blackberries	5,348	Tangerines	1,620
Raspberries	4,925	Russet potatoes (cooked)	1,555
Almonds	4,454	Red grapefruits	1,548
Red Delicious apples	4,275	Green cabbage	1,359
Green peas	4039	Red grapes	1,260
Chickpeas (garbanzo beans)	4,030	Broccoli (cooked)	1,259
Dates	3,895	Onions (yellow)	1,220
Strawberries	3,577	Carrots (raw)	1,215
Figs	3,383	Green grapes	1,118
Cherries	3,361	Mangoes	1,002

Antioxidant-rich drinks include green, black and white teas, plus red wine – the latter in moderation, please.

FLUSHING WITH FIBRE

Dietary fibre, or roughage, includes substances such as cellulose, hemicellulose, lignin, pectins and gums that pass through the small intestines undigested, as we human beings lack the enzymes needed to break them down.

There are two main types: soluble and insoluble fibre. Soluble fibre is most important in the stomach and upper intestines, where it mops up fats and sugars to slow the rate at which they pass into the circulation. Once fibre reaches the large bowel, enzymes released by bowel bacteria ferment it and break it down, releasing gases with various smelly odours (especially from beans). Insoluble fibre is most important in the large bowel, where it absorbs water, bacteria and toxins, and provides bulk to help us excrete stools faster.

All plant foods contain both soluble and insoluble fibre, though some sources are richer in one type than another. For example, oats and figs are rich in soluble fibre, while wheat and leafy vegetables are a good source of insoluble fibre.

Fibre binds cholesterol and other fats in the bowel to reduce their absorption and

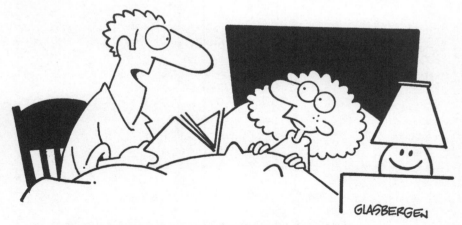

'First, Goldilocks ate Daddy Bear's porridge, then she ate
Mummy Bear's porridge, then she ate Baby Bear's porridge ...
and her cholesterol dropped 20%!'

can have a significant effect on cholesterol levels. Eating one bowl of oatmeal a day can reduce LDL-cholesterol by 8-23%. Taking 10g psyllium seed supplements (see page 38) daily for at least six weeks has also been shown to reduce 'bad' LDL-cholesterol levels by between 5 and 20%.

A healthy diet ideally provides at least 18g (0.6oz) fibre per day – around 40% higher than current average intakes. Levels of greater than 30g (1oz) per day are thought to be best for proper bowel function. In evolutionary terms, this level of intake is still low – our Stone-Age ancestors regularly ate over 100g (3.5oz) fibre per day from a variety of plant sources.

FOODS CONTAINING 3g OR MORE FIBRE PER 100g ARE HIGH-FIBRE CHOICES:

FOOD	Fibre per 100g
Bran	40g
Dried apricots	18g
Prunes	13g
Brown bread	6g
Walnuts	6g
Peas	5g
Cooked wholemeal spaghetti	4g

STEROLS AND STANOLS

Sterols and stanols have a similar chemical structure to cholesterol, and reduce absorption of dietary cholesterol by competing for the enzymes and receptors needed for its absorption. As a result, people with the highest dietary intake of plant sterols have the lowest cholesterol levels, as was shown in a large trial involving over 22,500 men and women living in Norfolk, UK. Eating 2g plant sterols or stanols per day can signifi-cantly lower LDL-cholesterol and help to protect against heart disease. However, the average diet supplies only between 160 and 460mg per day, with vegetarians obtaining the highest amounts. Functional foods fortified with sterols such as spreads and yoghurts have therefore been developed to boost levels. Including 20-25g (less than 1oz) of fortified spread in your diet can lower LDL-cholesterol by 10-15% within as little as three weeks.

When changing to a high-fibre diet, or taking fibre supplements, increase your intake gradually to prevent the feelings of bloating and distension that can occur during the first two to three weeks. It is also important to ensure you drink lots of fluids.

LOSING WEIGHT

If you have a high cholesterol level it is vitally important that you shed any excess weight. Losing 10kg/22lb will lower your blood pressure, reduce your blood glucose levels and improve cholesterol levels enough to reduce your overall risk of premature death by 20%. And getting down to the healthy weight range for your height can reduce your risk of a heart attack by over 50%.

FIND A TAPE MEASURE and check the size of your waist in centimetres. If it's greater than 80cm and you are female, or if it's larger than 94cm and you are male, then you are apple-shaped. Storing fat round your middle (central obesity) increases your risk of heart disease by 70% and your risk of developing type 2 diabetes by 80%.

Although low-fat diets are still recommended by traditional doctors and dieticians, they are no better than low-calorie diets (providing 1,200-1,500 kcals per day) in helping people achieve long-term weight-loss goals; it is the energy restriction that helps weight loss rather than the fact that the diet is low in fat. And, unfortunately, low-fat diets usually lower 'good' HDL-cholesterol levels by at least as much as they do 'bad' LDL-cholesterol. For most people, especially those who've inherited the type of metabolism associated with central obesity (see pages 8-9), a low glycaemic index (GI) diet is most effective. Low GI diets restrict your intake of the simple carbohydrates that raise blood glucose levels and trigger the secretion of insulin – the body's main fat-storing hormone. A low GI diet can help you lose weight, lower triglyceride and LDL-cholesterol levels and raise HDL-cholesterol.

The following chart shows healthy weight ranges for the average adult, according to height and sex. If your weight falls above the range given for your height, try to lose weight slowly and steadily until you fall within your healthy range.

OPTIMUM HEALTHY WEIGHT RANGE

HEIGHT Metres/Feet		MEN Kg/Stones		WOMEN Kg/Stones	
1.47	4'10"	43 – 54	6st 11lb – 8st 7lb	40 – 51	6st 4lb – 8st
1.50	4'11	45 – 56	7st 1lb – 8st 11lb	42 – 54	6st 8lb – 8st 7lb
1.52	5ft	46 – 58	7st 3lb – 9st 2lb	43 – 55	6st 11lb – 8st 9lb
1.55	5'1"	48 – 60	7st 8lb – 9st 7lb	45 – 57	7st 1lb – 8st 13lb
1.57	5'2"	49 – 62	7st 10lb – 9st 11lb	46 – 59	7st 3lb – 9st 4lb
1.60	5'3"	51 – 64	8st – 10st 1lb	48 – 61	7st 8lb – 9st 8lb
1.63	5'4"	53 – 66	8st 5lb – 10st 6lb	50 – 63	7st 12lb – 9st 13lb
1.65	5'5"	54 – 68	8st 7lb – 10st 10lb	51 – 65	8st – 10st 3lb
1.68	5'6"	56 – 70	8st 12lb – 11st	53 – 67	8st 5lb – 10st 7lb
1.70	5'7"	58 – 72	9st 1lb – 11st 4lb	54 – 69	8st 7lb – 10st 12lb
1.73	5'8"	60 – 75	9st 6lb – 11st 10lb	56 – 71	8st 11lb – 11st 2lb
1.75	5'9"	61 – 76	9st 9lb – 12st	57 – 73	8st 13lb – 11st 7lb
1.78	5'10"	63 – 79	9st 13lb – 12st 6lb	59 – 75	9st 4lb – 11st 11lb
1.80	5'11"	65 – 81	10st 3lb – 12st 9lb	61 – 77	9st 8lb – 12st 1lb
1.83	6ft	67 – 83	10st 7lb – 13st 1lb	63 – 80	9st 13lb – 12st 8lb
1.85	6'1"	69 – 85	10st 11lb – 13st 5lb		
1.88	6'2"	71 – 88	11st 2lb – 13st 12lb		
1.90	6'3"	72 – 90	11st 5lb – 14st 2lb		
1.93	6'4"	75 – 93	11st 10lb – 14st 8lb		

Based on a body mass index (BMI) of 18.7-23.8 for women, and a BMI of 20-25 for men.

EXERCISING CONTROL
Exercise increases your metabolic rate by as much as ten times, mobilizing fatty acids from your fat stores and increasing the rate at which they are burned for fuel in the muscle cells.

Bouts of exercise, such as brisk walking, cause blood-fat levels to rise much less than usual after a high-fat meal. This effect is noticeable when exercise is taken as much as 15 hours before a meal, or 90 minutes afterwards – and it's important because high blood-fat levels after eating are now recognized as one of the main triggers for atherosclerosis.

Perhaps the most striking example of how exercise affects blood fats was shown by Sir Ranulph Fiennes and Dr Michael Stroud during their epic, unassisted journey across the Antarctic in 1992. They ate over 5,500 kcals a day, including twice the amount of fat recommended (mostly in the form of butter), to provide as much energy as possible without increasing the weight of rations they had to carry. Regular blood tests showed their total blood-cholesterol levels did not change, but their level of beneficial HDL-cholesterol, which protects against coronary heart disease (CHD), went up while their level of harmful LDL-cholesterol went down.

Researchers believe that regular exercise reduces the amount of harmful very low-density lipoproteins (VLDL) and triglycerides produced by the liver. It also increases levels of an enzyme made by the muscles that breaks down cholesterol for use as a fuel (lipoprotein lipase). The good effect of exercise on blood-fat levels

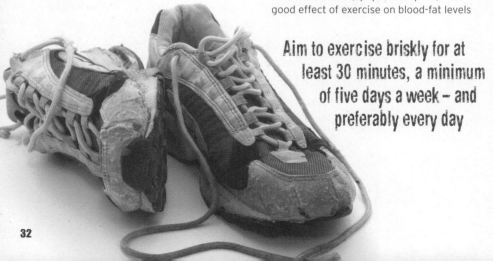

Aim to exercise briskly for at least 30 minutes, a minimum of five days a week – and preferably every day

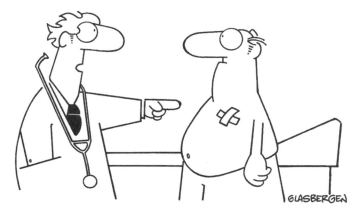

'Whenever your cholesterol goes too high,
a sensor will send a signal that automatically locks
the kitchen and turns on your treadmill.'

occurs with just a single bout of exercise, but the effect on muscle enzymes does not develop until the fifth regular session.

Long-distance runners have significantly lower concentrations of small, low-density lipoproteins and VLDLs while producing higher concentrations of beneficial HDLs than sedentary males. Fat levels in the blood of trained athletes are also 42% lower and fat is cleared 75% faster than usual. In addition, exercise lowers your blood pressure, improves the dilation of the arteries and improves glucose tolerance, as well as helping you lose excess weight. These beneficial effects are soon lost, however, if physical activity is stopped. The best thing, therefore: exercise on a daily basis.

As a result of all these beneficial effects, regular physical activity reduces your risk of death at any age for all causes, especially CHD, by 25%. Among those who exercise briskly for at least three hours a week, the risk of CHD was reduced by 30–40%. This is true even when other risk factors such as age, smoking habits, cholesterol levels, blood pressure, blood glucose levels and your family history of heart disease are taken into account.

Your goal is to exercise briskly for at least 30 minutes, on a minimum of five days a week – and preferably every day. If you are unfit, start off slowly and increase your effort as you become more fit. The 30 minutes of exercise do not even have to occur all in one go. Similar benefits on blood-fat levels are obtained from three 10-minute sessions per day, or two 15-minute sessions.

LIVING HEALTHILY
In addition to losing weight and exercising regularly, it is important that you stop smoking, keep your alcohol intake at sensible levels, avoid excess stress and find time for rest and relaxation.

SMOKING

Smokers are seven times more likely to have a heart attack and four times more likely to experience a stroke than non-smokers. The good news is that quitting can reduce your risk of these by as much as 50% within one year due to reduced blood stickiness, spasm and arterial constriction, lowered blood pressure, improved oxygenation of tissues and reduced likelihood of atherosclerosis.

Quitting isn't easy, but using nicotine replacement therapy (NRT) doubles your chance of success. Receiving behavioural counselling from a healthcare profes-sional in addition to NRT increases the likelihood of quitting by a further 26%.

The gradual reduction method is another useful option. This reduces your intake of nicotine by applying drops of a natural corn-syrup product onto cigarette

If you do smoke, consider taking pycnogenol (see page 37) – extracts from the bark of the French maritime pine – which is as effective in preventing blood clots in smokers as aspirin, but without irritating the stomach.

filters immediately before smoking. It is typically used over a six-week period to wean you gently from nicotine addiction and has a 60% success rate (go to www.nicobloc.com).

NRT is available as skin patches, lozenges, chewing-gum, inhalers, sprays and microtabs that dissolve in the mouth. Other drugs to aid smoking cessation are available on prescription.

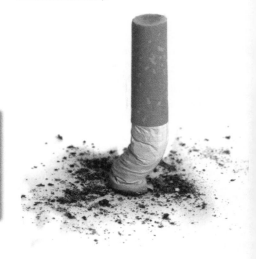

ALCOHOL

A light-to-moderate intake of alcohol (especially antioxidant-rich red wine) raises good HDL-cholesterol, lowers blood pressure and reduces the risk of coronary heart disease. It may also reduce abnormal blood-clotting and improve the state of your artery walls – think of it as a bit like paint-stripper, dissolving away some of the fatty buildup. Excess alcohol, however, raises triglyceride levels, pushes up blood pressure and increases the risk of heart attack, congestive heart failure and sudden death from abnormal heart rhythms. That's before we even mention the harmful effects on liver health. Balance is the key.

Men should not drink more than 3-4 units per day on a regular basis, while women should have no more than 2-3 drinks per day. Aim for two or more alcohol-free days per week, as well.

STRESS

Stress raises your blood pressure, lowers immunity and, according to new findings, raises cholesterol levels, too. People experiencing the most stress are three times more likely to have a raised LDL-cholesterol level than those experiencing the least amount of stress, even when taking other risk factors into account. This is because stress hormones such as adrenaline (epinephrine) and cortisol prepare the body for flight-or-fight by increasing the availability of circulating fuels (glucose, fatty acids, LDL) for the muscle cells.

WHEN FEELING STRESSED:

- Stop what you are doing and repeat a soothing mantra such as 'calm' inwardly to yourself.
- Concentrate on breathing slowly and deeply.
- Go for a brisk walk to burn off the effects of stress hormones.

LIFESTYLE CHANGE	REDUCTION IN RISK OF A HEART ATTACK WITHIN FIVE YEARS
Stopping smoking	50-70%
Losing excess weight	35-55%
Exercising for at least three hours a week	30-40%
Keeping alcohol intakes within healthy limits	25-45% lower risk than those who drink excessively

SUPER SUPPLEMENTS A number of
nutritional supplements can lower cholesterol levels or
slow the progression of atherosclerosis.

SUPPLEMENT	BENEFIT	DOSE
Vitamin C	Vitamin C is an antioxidant that protects against coronary heart disease. Research involving over 6,600 men and women found that those with the highest levels enjoyed a 27% lower risk of coronary heart disease and a 26% lower risk of stroke than those with low levels.	Usual dose: 250mg-2g daily
Vitamin E	Vitamin E is an antioxidant that protects circulating cholesterol and polyunsaturated fats from oxidation. The Cambridge Heart Antioxidant Study showed that taking high-dose vitamin E (at least 400iu daily) reduced the risk of a heart attack by as much as 77%. Other large trials have shown that both men and women can reduce their risk of ever developing coronary heart disease by as much as 40% through taking vitamin E supplements.	Usual dose: 100-400iu (around 67-268 mg) vitamin E per day, combined with other antioxidants such as vitamin C and selenium
Carotenoids	Carotenoids are yellow, orange and red antioxidant pigments (eg betacarotene, lycopene, lutein). Those with the highest carotenoid intakes are 50% less likely to develop coronary heart disease, and 75% less likely to experience a heart attack than those with low intakes.	Usual dose: 15mg mixed carotenoids
Selenium	Selenium is an antioxidant mineral, lack of which is associated with low HDL-cholesterol levels and an increased risk of atherosclerosis, heart attack and stroke. Low intakes of selenium are a growing cause for concern throughout most of Europe.	Usual dose: 50-200mcg daily

Vitamin B₃

Vitamin B₃, also known as niacin, or nicotinic acid, is important for the processing of fatty acids. It is prescribed to lower stubbornly high triglycerides and LDL-cholesterol levels, while increasing levels of good HDL-cholesterol. At high doses (under medical supervision) it reduces the risk of both fatal and non-fatal heart attacks.

Usual dose: 15–30mg in vitamin supplements. Higher prescription doses (500mg–2g daily) can produce facial flushing; low-dose aspirin taken half an hour beforehand can reduce this effect

Folic acid

Folic acid/folate is essential for the processing of homocysteine – an amino acid that triggers atherosclerosis. The type of folate found naturally in food sources such as green leafy vegetables is less easily absorbed and less active in the body than the synthetic version, folic acid, which you can get from supplements and fortified foods such as breakfast cereals.

Usual dose: 400–650mcg per day. Vitamins B₆ and B₁₂ also have a beneficial effect on homocysteine processing

Pycnogenol

Pycnogenol is extracted from the bark of the French maritime pine. It contains a variety of potent antioxidants that help to lower blood pressure, improve dilation of small blood vessels, reduce blood stickiness and slow the progression of atherosclerosis. It can significantly reduce LDL-cholesterol and increase HDL-cholesterol, and also reduces abnormal blood-clotting in smokers.

Usual dose: 50–200mg daily

Omega-3 fish oils

Omega-3 fish oils increase the ratio of beneficial HDL-cholesterol to LDL-cholesterol, and significantly lower triglyceride levels. They also reduce blood stickiness and abnormal heart rhythms. In those who have had a heart attack, omega-3 fish oils significantly reduce the chance of a second heart attack. If one does occur, the chance of dying from this second heart attack is significantly decreased.

Usual dose: 1.5–5g daily. Seek medical advice before taking if you have a blood-clotting disorder or are taking a blood-thinning drug such as warfarin

SUPER SUPPLEMENTS CONT.

SUPPLEMENT	BENEFIT	DOSE
Garlic	Garlic extracts have been shown in some studies to reduce LDL-cholesterol levels by an average of 11%. Evidence from 152 people followed for four years also suggests they reduce and even reverse hardening and furring-up of the arteries. In addition, garlic lowers blood pressure and improves arterial dilation.	**Usual dose:** 900mg daily
Lecithin	Lecithin (phosphatidyl choline) is a type of fat that inhibits intestinal absorption of cholesterol, and increases its excretion into the bile. Taking high-dose lecithin for 30 days can reduce average total cholesterol, LDL-cholesterol and triglycerides by over a third, while increasing beneficial HDL-cholesterol by 46%.	**Usual dose:** 1-10g daily. One hen's egg supplies around 2g lecithin
Isoflavones	Isoflavones are plant hormones extracted from soyabeans that have a weak, oestrogen-like action. They are especially helpful for post-menopausal women, helping to dilate coronary arteries, as well as reducing LDL-cholesterol and abnormal blood-clotting. Regular intake can lower total cholesterol and LDL-cholesterol by 4% or more. Research consistently shows an association between diets rich in these phytoestrogens, and a reduced risk of cardiovascular disease.	**Usual dose:** 25-50mg daily
Psyllium	Psyllium seeds and husks are a natural fibre source that binds cholesterol and other fats in the bowel. This slows their absorption so the body can handle them more easily. Taking 10g of psyllium seeds daily for at least six weeks can reduce 'bad' LDL-cholesterol levels by between 5 and 20%.	**Usual dose:** 1-10g daily; start with a small increase in fibre intake and slowly increase. Drink plenty of water

Probiotics

Probiotics are live, friendly bacteria that improve digestion and the immune system. They also produce short-chain fatty acids that act on the liver to reduce blood stickiness and lower raised cholesterol levels.

Usual dose:
1–2 billion colony-forming units (CFU)

Plant sterols

Plant sterols such as campesterol, sitosterol and stigmasterol closely resemble cholesterol. They block absorption of dietary cholesterol to reduce LDL-cholesterol levels by 15%. In those with type 2 diabetes, this effect is almost doubled (26.8% reduction). Adding plant sterols to statin medication is more effective than doubling the statin dose.

Usual dose:
1–2g daily

Red yeast rice

Red yeast rice is made by fermenting a type of yeast, *Monascus purpureus*, over rice, and is often used as a food colouring in dishes such as Peking duck. Red yeast rice is the Chinese medicine equivalent of a statin, lowering cholesterol in the same way by inhibiting the enzyme (HMG-CoA reductase) needed to synthesize cholesterol in the liver. It can reduce total cholesterol by 23%, LDL-cholesterol by 31% and triglycerides by 34% while increasing beneficial HDL-cholesterol by 20%. Recent research involving almost 5,000 adults who had previously experienced a heart attack found that taking red yeast rice extract for an average of 4.5 years reduced the risk of having another non-fatal heart attack and of dying from coronary heart disease by 45% compared with those taking a placebo. Some side effects in the muscles, similar to those seen with statin drugs, have been reported, however, so this supplement should also be combined with Coenzyme Q10.

Usual dose:
1.2–2.4g daily

Coenzyme Q10 should be considered by anyone taking a statin drug or a red yeast rice extract to offset muscle side effects (see pages 16–17). **Usual dose:** 60–120mg daily

LOWER YOUR

If you can lower your LDL-cholesterol and increase your HDL-cholesterol levels, you are less likely to experience a heart attack or stroke than if you don't.

WHY?

For every 1% reduction in your LDL-cholesterol level, your risk of cardio-vascular disease falls by 2%. In addition, for every 1% rise in beneficial HDL-cholesterol, your risk of cardiovascular disease is reduced by at least 2%.

WHERE ARE YOU NOW?

In order to monitor your progress, you need to know your current status. So before starting the 12-week cholesterol-reduction project, you should have your total cholesterol, LDL-cholesterol, HDL-cholesterol and triglyceride levels measured by your doctor, or done privately. Many pharmacies offer this as a health-screening service. As explained on pages 12–13, these blood tests are taken first thing in the morning, before eating or drinking.

It's also a good idea to have your current weight and blood pressure measured (record the results in the charts on page 54–55). If possible, also have your blood homocysteine level checked (see pages 12–13).

WHERE DO YOU WANT TO BE?

The general aim of any cholesterol-lowering regime is to lower your total cholesterol to less than 5mmol/l (200mg/dl) or by 30%, whichever is the greater.

Ideally, you want to lower your LDL-cholesterol to less than 3mmol/l (100mg/dl), and increase your HDL-cholesterol to greater than 1mmol/l (40mg/dl) for men, or 1.2mmol/l (50mg/dl) for women.

The lower your LDL the better, and the higher your HDL, the more protection you will have against the artery-narrowing disorder atherosclerosis.

In addition, if your triglycerides are raised, you want to bring them down to less than 1.7mmol/l (150mg/dl).

These are your goals. When you come to the end of the 12 weeks, retake the tests and work out your percentage improvements, and the amount by which you have lowered your risk of a heart attack and stroke.

CHOLESTEROL IN 12 WEEKS

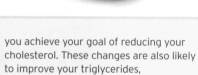

NB: BEFORE STARTING THE PROCESS, please buy yourself a simple step-counting pedometer that records the number of footsteps you take per day. These are readily available in sports shops or online, and cost very little.

HOW ARE YOU GOING TO GET THERE?

We are creatures of habit, and bad dietary and lifestyle habits are hard to break. To accomplish changes in the long term, you need to break things down into little, positive steps that are easier to introduce as new, permanent habits.

The Japanese have a useful philosophy, *kaizen* – committing yourself to making continuous, small steps towards improvement. This is the ideal approach to take if you want to improve your cholesterol balance.

Each week, your goal is to focus on a relatively small dietary change that will help to improve your LDLs and HDLs significantly. Each week also includes an exercise plan and lifestyle tip that will help

you achieve your goal of reducing your cholesterol. These changes are also likely to improve your triglycerides, homocysteine, blood pressure and weight.

After achieving each weekly dietary goal, you get to choose a reward to aid your motivation, such as a new book, DVD or CD, a manicure or facial, or a new DIY tool. Write your chosen reward in the allotted space for each week.

As you introduce each new change, be sure to maintain the old changes so that, by the end of the process, these new beneficial habits will have become second nature. The changes you make in the first few weeks will be more deeply ingrained than those made in the last few weeks, but, as you move forward in life, you will soon do them all without thinking.

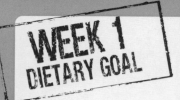

WEEK 1
DIETARY GOAL

EAT AT LEAST FIVE SERVINGS OF FRUIT AND VEGETABLES A DAY

Eat them raw, where appropriate, or only lightly steamed to obtain the greatest cholesterol-lowering benefits (see pages 26-27). For example, have:

Breakfast
A handful of berries or a chopped banana with your cereal, and/or half a grapefruit (check for drug interactions, eg with statins) plus a glass of (preferably freshly squeezed) orange juice

Mid-morning
An apple

Lunch
A large mixed salad and a pear

Dinner
A portion of spinach; some carrots and/or sweetcorn along with your protein (eg fish); plus a handful of grapes with dessert

EXERCISE PLAN Using your new best friend, your pedometer, which now goes everywhere with you, record the number of paces you take every day this week, without making any special effort to increase your activity level. Write the number of steps you take per day in the chart on pages 58-59. Total up the number of steps for the week, and divide by seven to obtain the average number of steps you have taken each day this week.

LIFESTYLE TIP Aim to maintain a healthy weight for your height. Use the chart on pages 30-31 to find out your ideal weight range and keep this in mind as your target. Lose any excess weight slowly and steadily rather than going for a quick fix and you're more likely to succeed. Filling in the chart on pages 58-59 will also help you stick with your new healthy lifestyle in the long term.

Tick the chart on pages 56-57 for every day that you achieve your minimum of five portions of fruit and veg this week – your vital '5-a-day'!

 MY REWARD FOR THIS WEEK IS: ....

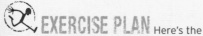
EAT MORE OILY FISH

Boys, men and women who are not planning on having more children should aim to eat three or four portions (115g/4oz each) of oily fish a week (see pages 22–23). If you are female and likely to have a child at some stage, aim to eat two portions of oily fish a week (the lower amount is to reduce exposure to potential marine pollutants).

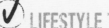

Write you target number of portions this week here: ....

EXERCISE PLAN Here's the first small step to health! Increase the number of paces you take this week by 10%. To do this, take the average number of paces you walked per day last week, and multiply this figure by 1.1 (round up or down to the nearest five steps). For example, if the average number of paces you walked per day last week was 3,505, multiply this by 1.1 to obtain your total for this week of 3,855 paces or more per day. Your ultimate aim is to reach 10,000 paces or more per day by the end of the 12 weeks (though it may take you a bit longer if you start lower). Using the chart on pages 58–59 will help you reach this goal.

LIFESTYLE TIP Use healthier cooking methods. Steam, grill, boil, bake, poach or stir-fry foods rather than deep-frying. If roasting meat, place it on a rack within the roasting pan so the fats drain away. Roast potatoes with just a light brushing of olive oil.

PREVIOUS DIETARY GOALS TO MAINTAIN

- Continue to eat at least five servings of fruit and vegetables every day

Tick the chart on pages 56–57 for every day that you eat a portion of oily fish this week.

 MY REWARD FOR THIS WEEK IS: ....

EAT LESS SALT

Following a high-salt diet is linked with low levels of beneficial HDL-cholesterol. A high salt intake can also increase blood pressure. Obtain flavour instead from garlic, fresh herbs and spices, freshly ground black pepper and more garlic (see page 19). Don't add table salt to food during cooking or at the table, and avoid obviously salty foods such as crisps, as well as foods that contain more salt than you might think – including cereal.

Check labels
If the salt content is given as 'sodium', multiply by 2.5 to obtain the salt (sodium chloride) content. For example, a product containing 0.4g sodium contains 1g of salt. A good rule of thumb is that, per 100g/3.5oz food (or per serving if a serving is less than 100g), 0.5g sodium or more is a lot of sodium; 0.1g sodium or less is a little.

EXERCISE PLAN
Again, increase your number of paces this week by 10%. Take the average number of paces you walked per day last week, and multiply by 1.1 (round up or down to the nearest five steps). For example, if the average number of paces you walked per day last week was 3,855, multiply this by 1.1 to obtain your new target of 4,240 paces or more per day. Use the chart on pages 58–59 to record your daily paces. Seeing the improvement will encourage you to stay focused.

LIFESTYLE TIP
If you smoke, do your utmost to stop. The chart on pages 58–59 will help you achieve your goal.

PREVIOUS DIETARY GOALS TO MAINTAIN
- Eat your '5-a-day' at least
- Eat more oily fish

Tick the chart on pages 56–57 for every day that you reduce your salt intake this week.

MY REWARD FOR THIS WEEK IS: ....

WEEK 4
DIETARY GOAL

EAT LESS TRANS FAT

Get into the habit of checking the labels on all the foods that you buy, and select only those with the lowest levels of trans fats or partially hydrogenated polyunsaturated fats (see pages 24-25).

EXERCISE PLAN Aim to increase the number of paces you take this week by another 10%. Once again, take the average number of paces you walked per day last week, and multiply by 1.1. So if the average number of paces you walked per day last week was 4,240, multiply this by 1.1 to obtain your new daily target of 4,665 paces or more. To help you stick with it, rather than see it as a chore, try to enjoy your walking time and see it as a period of stress-busting reflection. Choose routes you will look forward to walking, perhaps where the gardens have the prettiest flowers, or there's less traffic, or see it as a chance to give your dog more exercise as well, if you have one. Use the chart on pages 58-59 to record your daily paces.

 LIFESTYLE TIP Keep your alcohol intake within safe limits (see pages 34-35). And consider switching to red wine if you don't already drink it, for its proven heart-health benefits.

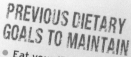

PREVIOUS DIETARY GOALS TO MAINTAIN
- Eat your '5-a-day' at least
- Eat more oily fish
- Eat less salt

Tick the chart on pages 56-57 for every day that you consciously avoid trans fats or partially hydrogenated polyunsaturated fats.

 MY REWARD FOR THIS WEEK IS: ....

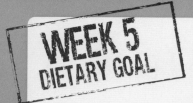

WEEK 5 DIETARY GOAL

EAT LESS SATURATED FAT AND PRE-FORMED CHOLESTEROL

We need to start getting strict now. Avoid processed meats and offal, and decrease the amount of red meat you eat to no more than three meals per week. Trim visible fat from meat. Switch to omega-3-enriched eggs, and limit yourself to three a week (see the chart on pages 20-21).

Use skimmed or semi-skimmed rather than whole-milk products, and use low-fat versions of as many foods as possible, eg mayonnaise, yoghurts, salad dressings, cheese etc.

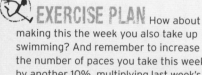**EXERCISE PLAN** How about making this the week you also take up swimming? And remember to increase the number of paces you take this week by another 10%, multiplying last week's average by 1.1. So if you walked an average of 4,665 last week, multiply this by 1.1 to obtain your new daily target of 5,130 paces this week. Use the chart on pages 58-59 to record your daily paces.

- An antioxidant supplying additional vitamins C and E, carotenoids and selenium
- Omega-3 fish oils
- Folic acid
- Pycnogenol (especially if you smoke)
- Coenzyme Q10 (especially if you are taking a statin drug; see pages 14-17)

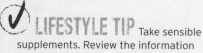**LIFESTYLE TIP** Take sensible supplements. Review the information on pages 36-39 and decide which supplements are right for you. I suggest:

PREVIOUS DIETARY GOALS TO MAINTAIN

- Eat your '5-a-day' at least
- Eat more oily fish
- Eat less salt
- Eat less trans fat

Tick the chart on pages 56-57 for every day that you consciously eat fewer foods containing saturated fat or pre-formed cholesterol this week.

 MY REWARD FOR THIS WEEK IS: ....

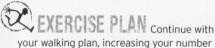

WEEK 6 DIETARY GOAL

EAT MORE VEGETARIAN MEALS

In place of red meat, eat more beans, lentils and peas for protein. These are also good sources of soluble fibre. Eating 200g/7oz of cooked beans a day can lower LDL-cholesterol by 15-20% in just a month. Experiment with soyabeans, black-eyed peas, Puy lentils, red lentils, butterbeans, chickpeas (garbanzo beans), green beans, kidney beans, lima beans, pinto beans, adzuki beans – the range is immense. They make wonderful soups, curries, stews, casseroles and pasta sauces when combined with tomatoes, onions, garlic, spices and herbs. Buy a vegetarian cookbook – or find millions of free recipes online.

EXERCISE PLAN Continue with your walking plan, increasing your number of paces by another 10% (multiply last week's figure by 1.1). So if your average number of paces last week was 5,130, multiply this by 1.1 to get your new target of 5,645 paces per day this week. Use the chart on pages 58-59 to record your progress. In addition, check out the lifestyle advice on other types of exercise below.

LIFESTYLE TIP Now that you are relatively fit and may be achieving over 5,000 paces per day, start engaging in at least 30 minutes of additional moderate-to-vigorous physical activity per day, if you are not already doing so. Try cycling, dancing, jogging, football or racquet sports. Exercise is one of the best ways to cut cholesterol (see pages 32-33).

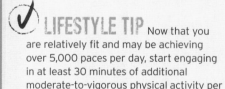

PREVIOUS DIETARY GOALS TO MAINTAIN

- Eat your '5-a-day' at least
- Eat more oily fish
- Eat less salt
- Eat less trans fat
- Eat less saturated fat and pre-formed cholesterol

Tick the chart on pages 56-57 for every day that you follow a vegetarian diet this week (aim for three if you can).

 MY REWARD FOR THIS WEEK IS: ....

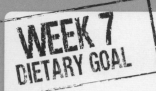

WEEK 7
DIETARY GOAL

EAT MORE
WHOLE GRAINS

As well as providing important cholesterol-lowering vitamins and minerals, the fibre in whole grains reduces the amount of dietary cholesterol you absorb. Choose brown rice, wholemeal bread and wholewheat pasta in place of less healthy 'white' versions, and experiment with hemp pasta (made from hemp-seed flour), red rice, wild rice (the seed of a water grass), buckwheat and quinoa (the seed of a plant related to spinach).

 EXERCISE PLAN Are you enjoying your daily walks? Would you miss them if you cut down or dropped them altogether? If so, it's a sure sign that all this exercise is starting to have a positive effect! Once again, increase the number of paces you take this week by 10%, multiplying last week's figure by 1.1. So if last week's average number of paces per day was 5,645, multiply this by 1.1 to obtain your new target of 6,210 daily paces or more this week. Doesn't it feel good to know that your daily step count has come on so far already? Use the chart on pages 58–59 to help you record your daily paces.

 LIFESTYLE TIP Take time out for regular rest and relaxation. Meditation and yoga have both been shown to lower high cholesterol levels and reduce harmful oxidation of circulating fats.

PREVIOUS DIETARY GOALS TO MAINTAIN

- Eat your '5-a-day' at least
- Eat more oily fish
- Eat less salt
- Eat less trans fat
- Eat less saturated fat and pre-formed cholesterol
- Eat more vegetarian meals

Tick the chart on pages 56–57 for every day that you eat more whole grains this week.

 MY REWARD FOR THIS WEEK IS: ....

EAT MORE NUTS AND SEEDS

These are rich sources of beneficial omega-3s and monounsaturated fatty acids (see pages 24-25). Aim to eat a handful of almonds, Brazils, hazelnuts, macadamias, pistachios or walnuts per day. Use nut oils in salad dressings, and sprinkle a handful of mixed seeds over cereals, salads, vegetables, desserts – anything!

EXERCISE PLAN The great news is that you're getting closer to that 10,000 a day target! Increase the number of paces you take this week by another 10%. So if your average number of daily paces last week was 6,210, multiply this by 1.1 to obtain your new target this week of 6,830 paces per day or more. Use the chart on pages 58-59 to record just how far you've advanced.

LIFESTYLE TIP Drink more tea. Green, black and white teas contain powerful antioxidants that block cholesterol absorption and increase excretion of cholesterol-containing bile. Tea antioxidants also increase the breakdown of triglycerides. Compared with non-tea drinkers, those enjoying 4-5 cups of tea a day are half as likely to have a heart attack or stroke. And increase your intake of 70%-cocoa dark chocolate – it's packed with antioxidants.

PREVIOUS DIETARY GOALS TO MAINTAIN
- Eat your '5-a-day' at least
- Eat more oily fish
- Eat less salt
- Eat less trans fats
- Eat less saturated fat and pre-formed cholesterol
- Eat more vegetarian meals
- Eat more whole grains

Tick the chart on pages 56-57 for every day that you eat a handful of nuts and seeds this week.

 MY REWARD FOR THIS WEEK IS: ....

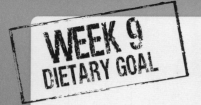

WEEK 9
DIETARY GOAL

EAT MORE FOODS FORTIFIED WITH PLANT STEROLS/STANOLS

As explained on pages 28-29, eating 20-25g (just less than 1oz) of fortified spread per day can lower LDL-cholesterol by 10-15% within as little as three weeks - perfect for the final three weeks of your cholesterol-reduction project. Look for spreads, yoghurts and other products fortified with these gems, too.

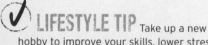

EXERCISE PLAN Do you look forward now to walking? If so, the good news is it's time to increase the number of paces you take this week by another 10%. So, if your average number of paces last week was 6,830 per day, multiply this by 1.1 to obtain your new target of 7,515 or more daily paces this week. Remember to use the chart on pages 58-59 to record how you're getting on.

LIFESTYLE TIP Take up a new hobby to improve your skills, lower stress levels, meet new people and increase your self-esteem. Hobbies such as gardening and DIY increase your activity

levels, too. People with a regular hobby tend to have a higher level of beneficial HDL-cholesterol.

PREVIOUS DIETARY GOALS TO MAINTAIN
- Eat your '5-a-day' at least
- Eat more oily fish
- Eat less salt
- Eat less trans fat
- Eat less saturated fat and pre-formed cholesterol
- Eat more vegetarian meals
- Eat more whole grains
- Eat more nuts and seeds

Tick the chart on pages 56-57 for every day that you eat a product fortified with plant sterols or stanols this week.

 MY REWARD FOR THIS WEEK IS: ....

WEEK 10 DIETARY GOAL

EAT FEWER OMEGA-6s

The changes made in the previous weeks have automatically lowered your intake of omega-6s. A certain amount is important for health, and you are obtaining adequate quantities from whole grains, pulses, nuts, seeds and sterol/stanol-fortified spreads. It's now time, though, to cut out unnecessary omega-6s, found in processed foods, convenience foods and manufactured goods. And if you're using safflower, sunflower or cornseed oils for cooking, please now switch to olive oil or rapeseed oil.

 EXERCISE PLAN Add another 10% of steps to your current tally. Can you notice the difference? Do you get out of breath less easily? Once again, take the average number of paces you walked per day last week, and multiply by 1.1. So if you walked 7,515 steps per day last week, your new daily target is 8,265 paces or more this week. Use the chart on pages 58-59 to record your daily paces.

 LIFESTYLE TIP Reduce stress levels (see page 35). Organize your life to manage your time more effectively – prioritize tasks and deal with pressures one at a time. Be assertive and say 'no' to unreasonable demands. Listen to calming background music to unwind.

PREVIOUS DIETARY GOALS TO MAINTAIN

- Eat your '5-a-day' at least
- Eat more oily fish
- Eat less salt
- Eat less trans fat
- Eat less saturated fat and pre-formed cholesterol
- Eat more vegetarian meals
- Eat more whole grains
- Eat more nuts and seeds
- Eat more foods fortified with sterols/stanols

Tick the chart on pages 56-57 for every day that you consciously eat fewer omega-6s this week.

🏆 **MY REWARD FOR THIS WEEK IS:** ....

EAT MORE HIGH-ORAC FRUIT AND VEG

You've eaten at least five (and preferably eight to ten) servings of fruit and vegetables since the first day of the cholesterol-reduction project. I'd now like you to concentrate on eating those with the highest antioxidant scores – see page 27 for the ORAC scores of different foods. Aim to consume 20,000 ORAC units per day, or more.

EXERCISE PLAN You may almost be in the home straight now. Increase the number of paces you take this week by another 10% and savour the fact that you've almost reached your target figure. If the average number of paces you walked per day last week was 8,265, multiply this by 1.1 to obtain your new daily target of 9,090 or more paces this week. One again, use the chart on pages 58–59 to record your daily paces.

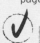

LIFESTYLE TIP Think positively. Researchers have found that people with an optimistic approach to life live 7.5 years longer than those with a gloomy outlook. Smile! Hug more! Make a point of complementing others around you – if you make them feel good about themselves, you'll enjoy the positive effects, too.

PREVIOUS DIETARY GOALS TO MAINTAIN

- Eat your '5-a-day' at least
- Eat more oily fish
- Eat less salt
- Eat less trans fat
- Eat less saturated fat and pre-formed cholesterol
- Eat more vegetarian meals
- Eat more whole grains
- Eat more nuts and seeds
- Eat more foods fortified with sterols/stanols
- Eat fewer omega-6s

Tick the chart on pages 56–57 for every day that you achieve your minimum of 20,000 ORAC units this week.

MY REWARD FOR THIS WEEK IS: ....

RELAX!

There are no more changes to make. You have now successfully taken the steps needed to reduce your cholesterol. Your task from now on is to maintain all the goals you've made so far, to help imprint them more firmly into your mind.

CONTINUE TO:

- Eat your '5-a-day' at least
- Eat more oily fish
- Eat less salt
- Eat less trans fat
- Eat less saturated fat and pre-formed cholesterol
- Eat more vegetarian meals
- Eat more whole grains
- Eat more nuts and seeds
- Eat more foods fortified with sterols/stanols
- Eat fewer omega-6s
- Eat more high-ORAC fruit and veg

EXERCISE PLAN By now you should be walking everywhere without giving it a second thought. Increase the number of paces you take this week by another 10%. Therefore, if the average number of paces you walked per day last week was 9,090, multiply this by 1.1 to obtain your new daily target of 10,000 paces or more. If so, you've reached the magical number of daily paces recommended for long-term health, in a period of just 12 weeks. Well done! (If you're not quite there yet, carry on increasing your steps till you do get there – it won't be long now.)

REASSESS Have your total, LDL- and HDL-cholesterol levels measured again, along with your triglycerides, blood pressure, waist measurement and weight. Record these figures in the charts on pages 54–55 and calculate your improvements.

YOUR REWARD Tick the chart on pages 56–57 for every day that you achieve all your dietary goals this week. The major reward for finishing this project is: A HOLIDAY. YOU DESERVE IT. But don't let those old, bad, eating and lifestyle habits creep back in. Visit a health spa rather than a resort featuring rich, gourmet foods.

CHOLESTEROL CHARTS

The general aim of any cholesterol-lowering process is to reduce your total cholesterol to less than 5mmol/l (200mg/dl) or by 30%, whichever is greater. Ideally, you want your LDL-cholesterol to be less than 3mmol/l (100mg/dl), and your HDL-cholesterol to be greater than 1mmol/l (40mg/dl) for men, or 1.2mmol/l (50mg/dl) for women. The lower your LDLs and the higher your HDLs, the better your atherosclerosis protection.

If your triglycerides are raised, you ideally want to bring them down to less than 1.7mmol/l (150mg/dl).

Ask your doctor what your target total cholesterol, HDL-cholesterol and LDL-cholesterol levels are and write them here:

MY TARGET total cholesterol level ....

MY TARGET HDL-cholesterol level ....

MY TARGET LDL-cholesterol level ....

THESE ARE YOUR GOALS Write your starting values in column **A**. When you finish the 12-week project, retake the tests and write your final values in column **B**. (See opposite for how to work out the percentage differences.)

Measurement	Optimal	A Start date	B End date	Percentage (%) change
Total cholesterol	Less than 5mmol/l (200mg/dl)			
LDL-cholesterol	Less than 3mmol/l (100mg/dl)			
HDL-cholesterol	Greater than: 1mmol/l (40 mg/dl) men; 1.2mmol/l (50mg/dl) women			
Triglycerides	Less than 1.7mmol/l (150mg/dl)			

WORKING OUT YOUR PERCENTAGE IMPROVEMENTS

To work out your percentage improvements, take the figure in column **A** and subtract the figure in column **B** (A-B).

Now, take the result of A-B and divide it by A, then multiply by 100.

$$\frac{A-B \times 100}{A} = X\%$$

So, if your initial LDL-cholesterol was 4.5 and your final figure is 3.1, it looks like this:

$$\frac{4.5-3.1 \times 100}{4.5} = 31.1\%$$

For every 1% reduction in your level of LDL-cholesterol, your risk of cardio-vascular disease reduces by 2%. So in this example you have reduced your risk of a heart attack or stroke by over 60%! And for every 1% RISE in beneficial HDL-cholesterol, your risk of cardiovascular disease falls by another 2%.

Please contact me, via my website, www.naturalhealthguru.co.uk, to let me know how you've got on.

MONITORING OTHER IMPORTANT FACTORS

Monitor your weight and blood pressure regularly. If you need to lose weight, use the chart on pages 58-59. Once you've achieved the healthy weight range for your height, don't let your weight increase by more than 1kg (2.2lb) without taking steps to reduce it.

If your blood pressure is consistently in the hypertensive range (140/90mmHg or more) seek advice from your doctor.

YOU MAY FIND THE FOLLOWING CHART USEFUL

Remember, your doctor is there to help. If, despite your best efforts, your health profile is not improving as well as you wish, seek professional advice.

		Date	Date	Date	Date	Date
MEASUREMENT	**TARGET**					
Weight	Within the healthy range for your height					
Waist measurement	Less than 80cm for women; less than 94cm for men					
Blood pressure	Less than 140/90 and preferably less than 130/80					

REWARD CHARTS

WEEK DAY/GOAL	1 EAT MORE FRUIT & VEG	2 EAT MORE OILY FISH	3 EAT LESS SALT	4 EAT LESS TRANS FAT	5 EAT LESS SATURATED FAT AND CHOLESTEROL	6 EAT MORE VEGETARIAN MEALS
Monday						
Tuesday						
Wednesday						
Thursday						
Friday						
Saturday						
Sunday						

WEEK COMPLETED REWARD STAR Colour in or stick on a gold star

★	★	★	★	★	★

**MY CHOSEN
REWARD FOR
THIS WEEK IS:**

Give yourself a tick in the following boxes for every day on which you successfully complete that week's task. Once you reach your target number of ticks for that week, you earn a gold star and can access the weekly reward you promised yourself!

WEEK DAY/GOAL	7 EAT MORE WHOLE GRAINS	8 EAT MORE NUTS & SEEDS	9 EAT MORE PLANT STEROLS/ STANOLS	10 EAT FEWER OMEGA-6S	11 EAT MORE HIGH-ORAC FOODS	12 MAINTAIN PREVIOUS DIETARY GOALS
Monday						
Tuesday						
Wednesday						
Thursday						
Friday						
Saturday						
Sunday						
WEEK COMPLETED REWARD STAR Colour in or stick on a gold star						
★	★	★	★	★	★
MY CHOSEN REWARD FOR THIS WEEK IS:						A holiday!

HEALTH CHARTS

Please record the average number of steps you take per day and week here.

Divide each weekly total by 7 to obtain the average number of paces taken per day for that week.

Increase the number of steps you aim to walk by 10% each week (just multiply by a factor of 1.1 to obtain your new target for the following week).

The last column gives you my suggested minimum number of daily steps to help you gradually increase to the target of 10,000 paces per day over the 12-week project.

CHART: PACES WALKED PER DAY

WEEK	Day 1	Day 2	Day 3	Day 4	Day 5	Day 6	Day 7	Weekly Total	Total divided by 7	Total multiplied by 1.1	Suggested Minimum
1											3,505
2											3,855
3											4,240
4											4,665
5											5,130
6											5,645
7											6,210
8											6,830
9											7,515
10											8,265
11											9,090
12											10,000

WEIGHT LOSS

Turn to the chart on pages 30-31 to find out the healthy weight range for your height.

MY TARGET weight range is:

.... to ....

If you are at the top end of the range, consider trying to lose a few pounds/kilos to get to further down your range. Aim to lose weight slowly and steadily, at a rate of 0.5–1kg (1-2lb) per week, by eating smaller portions and increasing your general level of activity. The 12-week cholesterol-reduction project will help you to eat more healthily overall. At the end of the 12 weeks, you may have lost at least 5.5k (12lb) of excess fat.

CHART: RECORD YOUR WEIGHT

WEEK	Weight	Amount of weight lost
1		
2		
3		
4		
5		
6		
7		
8		
9		
10		
11		
12		

CHART: QUIT SMOKING

Take it one day at a time. Record the number of cigarettes smoked each day, or tick off each cigarette-free day. Your goal is to have quit smoking by the end of week 12.

DAY	1	2	3	4	5	6	7
WEEK 1							
2							
3							
4							
5							
6							
7							
8							
9							
10							
11							
12							

QUIT TIPS

- Throw away all your cigarettes, lighters and smoking paraphernalia.
- Ask your doctor or pharmacist about nicotine replacement products, or use the gradual reduction method (see page 34).
- Occupy your hands with sketching, painting, knitting, DIY or origami to help break the hand-to-mouth habit
- Avoid situations where you used to smoke.

RESOURCES

GLOSSARY

Antioxidant A protective substance that helps to neutralize damaging oxidation reactions in the body, which are linked with premature ageing and disease.

Arcus senilis A premature yellow-white ring around the coloured part of the eyes.

Atherosclerosis Hardening and furring-up of the arteries.

Bile A yellow-green fluid made in the liver that is needed to digest fats.

Blood lipids Refers to total cholesterol, triglycerides and HDL- and LDL-cholesterol circulating in the blood; the blood test that measures these factors.

Carotenoid Orange-yellow antioxidant pigments found in fruit and vegetables.

CHD Coronary heart disease in which arteries supplying blood to the heart muscle are blocked by a buildup of plaque.

Cholesterol A waxy type of fat found in some animal foods and made in the body, mainly in the liver.

Coenzyme Q10 An enzyme needed for normal production of energy in body cells.

CRP C-reactive protein, a natural substance found in the blood that shows how much inflammation is present in the body. This includes the low-grade inflammation associated with a raised cholesterol level and atherosclerosis.

Essential fatty acids Dietary fats necessary for health, which cannot be made in the body but must come from food or supplements.

Fat Oily, organic compounds that don't dissolve in water but do dissolve in other oils; also known as lipids.

Free radicals Harmful unstable molecules created as part of normal metabolism. Excess free radicals can damage cells through a process called oxidation.

HDL High-density lipoprotein cholesterol. Also known as 'good' cholesterol, a type of lipoprotein that protects against atherosclerosis by carrying cholesterol back to the liver for processing.

HMG Co-A reductase 3-hydroxy-3-methyl-glutaryl Coenzyme A reductase, the enzyme involved in cholesterol synthesis, especially in the liver, that is blocked by the action of statin drugs.

Homocysteine An amino acid that can damage artery walls and hasten atherosclerosis. High levels of homocysteine are associated with an increased risk of coronary heart disease.

Hypercholesterolaemia A raised total blood cholesterol level.

Hypertension A raised blood pressure in which blood flows through the arteries with more force than normal.

Isoflavones Plant substances that have a weak oestrogen-like hormone action in the body. Present in high concentrations in soya extracts.

LDL Low-density lipoprotein cholesterol. Also known as 'bad' cholesterol as high levels are linked with atherosclerosis.

Lipids A general term for fats in the body.

Monounsaturated fat Dietary fat with one missing hydrogen atom; found in foods such as olive oil, nuts, seeds and avocados.

Omega-3 fatty acids A form of polyunsaturated dietary fat found in fish oil, flaxseed oil, walnut oil and some other vegetable oils.

Omega-6 fatty acids A form of polyunsaturated dietary fat found in many vegetable oils such as sunflower oil, safflower oil and corn oil.

ORAC Oxygen Radical Absorbance Capacity – a test that measures the antioxidant capacity of fruit and vegetable extracts.

Oxidation A chemical reaction that combines a substance with oxygen, similar to the process of rusting in metal.

Partially hydrogenated vegetable oil See Trans fat.

Plaque A porridge-like buildup of cholesterol and other substances on artery linings, leading to narrowing; plaque is formed in the process of atherosclerosis.

Platelets Cell fragments involved in blood-clotting.

Polyunsaturated fat Dietary fat that is missing more than one hydrogen atom; high amounts are present in corn and soyabean oil.

Probiotics the use of natural 'friendly' lactic acid-producing bacteria to encourage a healthy digestive balance and boost the immunity.

Saturated fat Dietary fat that contains as many hydrogen atoms as possible, such as is found in palm and coconut oil. Usually solid at room temperature.

Statins Drugs such as atorvastatin, pravastatin, fluvastatin, rosuvastatin and simvastatin that block the production of cholesterol within the body to lower total and LDL cholesterol.

Trans fat Partially hydrogenated or hydrogenated vegetable oil; a manufactured form of fat widely used in baked goods, fried foods and snack foods, which increases the risk of coronary heart disease.

Triglycerides Fats that circulate in the bloodstream and are stored as body fat. Elevated levels are an independent risk factor for heart disease.

Unsaturated fat Dietary fat that has some unfilled hydrogen bonds; includes polyunsaturated and monounsaturated fats.

VLDL Very low-density lipoprotein – a form of LDL-cholesterol that is associated with an increased risk of heart disease.

Xanthelasma Yellowish fatty lumps found in the skin around the eyes of some people with a very raised cholesterol level.

Xanthoma Fatty deposits in the tendon sheaths around the knees, elbows, fingers or heels of some people with a very raised cholesterol level.

USEFUL WEBSITES

Visit www.naturalhealthguru.co.uk to read more health information from Dr Sarah Brewer. You can also email me via this site to let me know how well you've succeeded by following the advice in the book.

CHOLESTEROL AND CIRCULATORY HEALTH

American Heart Association: www.americanheart.org
American Hypertension Society: www.ash-us.org
American Stroke Association: www.strokeassociation.org
Canadian Hypertension Society: www.hypertension.ca
Heart and Stroke Foundation of Canada:
www.heartandstroke.ca
Blood Pressure Association (UK): www.bpassoc.org.uk
British Heart Foundation: www.bhf.org.uk
British Hypertension Society: www.bhsoc.org
European Society of Hypertension: www.eshonline.org
Heart UK, the cholesterol charity: www.heartuk.org.uk
Consensus Action on Salt and Health (CASH):
www.hyp.ac.uk/cash

DIET

American Dietetic Association: www.eatright.org
United States Department of Agriculture's Food and Nutrition Information Center: www.nutrition.gov
Dieticians of Canada: www.dietitians.ca
British Nutrition Foundation: www.nutrition.org.uk
The Nutrition Society: www.nutritionsociety.org
British Dietetic Association: www.bda.uk.com

SMOKING

The Foundation for a Smokefree America:
www.anti-smoking.org
Action on Smoking and Health US: www.ash.org
Action on Smoking and Health Canada: www.ash.ca
Action on Smoking and Health UK: www.ash.org.uk
Quit UK www.quit.org.uk

ALCOHOL

National Institute on Alcohol Abuse and Alcoholism:
www.niaaa.nih.gov
Alcohol Concern: www.alcoholconcern.org.uk
Drink Aware Trust: www.drinkaware.co.uk

HERBAL MEDICINE

American Herbal Pharmacopoeia: www.herbal-ahp.org
American Herbalists Guild: www.americanherbalistsguild.com
International Register of Consultant Herbalists and Homeopaths: www.irch.org
UK National Institute of Medical Herbalists: www.nimh.org.uk

Quercus Editions Ltd
21 Bloomsbury Square
London WC1A 2NS

First Published 2009

Concept, text, design and layout © Quercus Editions Ltd 2009
The picture credits constitute an extension to this copyright notice.

A catalogue record for this book is available from the British Library.

ISBN: 978-1-84724-728-5

Printed in China

Every effort has been made to contact copyright holders. However, the publishers will be glad to rectify in future editions any inadvertent omissions brought to their attention.

Text by Dr Sarah Brewer
Edited by Ali Moore
Designed by Jane McKenna

Picture credits

Cartoons © Randy Glasbergen 5, 6, 10, 16, 28 and 33; iStockphoto/Ivan Montero 7, 23 (top), 25 and 35; iStockphoto 9; Science photo library/Victor De Schwanberg 12; Science photo library/James King-Holmes 15; iStockphoto/Paul Turner 18; iStockphoto/Stefanie Timmermann 19 (top); iStockphoto 19 (centre); iStockphoto/Jacob Wackerhausen 19 (bottom); iStockphoto 20; iStockphoto/Mark Jensen 23 (bottom); iStockphoto 24; Stockphoto 29; iStockphoto/Feng Yu 30; iStockphoto/Nicholas Monu 32; iStockphoto/Hermann Danzmayr 34; iStockphoto/Craig Veltri 41; iStockphoto 42-53